SAFETY FIRST

Safety in
Public Places

Joanne Mattern
ABDO Publishing Company

visit us at
www.abdopub.com

Published by Abdo Publishing Company 4940 Viking Drive, Edina, Minnesota 55435.
Copyright © 1999 by Abdo Consulting Group, Inc. International copyrights reserved in all
countries. No part of this book may be reproduced in any form without written permission
from the publisher.

Printed in the United States.

Photo credits: Peter Arnold, Inc., Super Stock

Edited by Julie Berg
Contributing editor Morgan Hughes
Graphics by Linda O'Leary

Library of Congress Cataloging-in-Publication Data

Mattern, Joanne, 1963-
    Safety in public places / Joanne Mattern.
    p. cm. -- (Safety first)
    Includes index.
    Summary: Suggests ways to put safety first when in public places such as
libraries, parks, stores, offices, busy streets, and neighborhoods.
    ISBN 1-57765-074-3
    1. Safety education--Juvenile literature. 2. Accidents--Prevention--Juvenile
literature. [1. Safety.] I. Title. II. Series.
    HQ770.7.M33   1999
    613.6--dc21   98-13897
                                          CIP
                                          AC

Contents

Safety First!

Public places are fun to visit! There are libraries and parks. There are stores and offices. There are busy streets to cross and neighborhoods to explore.

Wherever you go, it is important to always stay safe. Staying safe means you won't get hurt. You won't get in trouble. And you will keep other people from getting hurt or in trouble, too!

How can you stay safe in public places? The best way is to follow the rules and think before you act. This book will show you how to put safety first when you are in public places.

Opposite page:
You can have fun in public
places and stay safe, too.

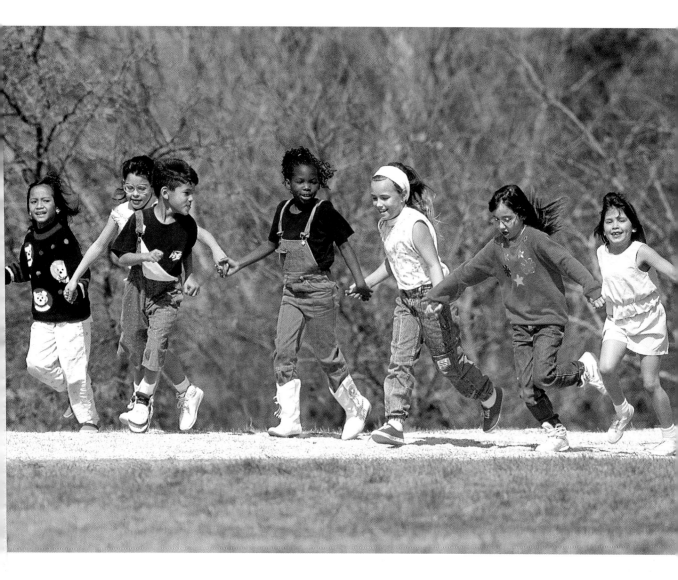

Traffic Lights

Traffic lights and signs are there to keep you safe. You will often see a traffic light at an **intersection** where two roads cross each other. A green light means go. A yellow light means go slowly and carefully. A red traffic light means stop. Cars have to obey these traffic lights. You should, too!

Some streets have lit-up signs that say "Walk" and "Don't Walk." These signs work with traffic lights to keep people and cars moving safely. If the "Don't Walk" sign is flashing, it means the light will soon turn red. Don't cross the street if the "Don't Walk" sign is flashing.

Always be sure to cross at the corner. A **crosswalk** is a safe place to walk. The middle of the street is not a safe place. It is against the law to cross there. You could even get a traffic ticket!

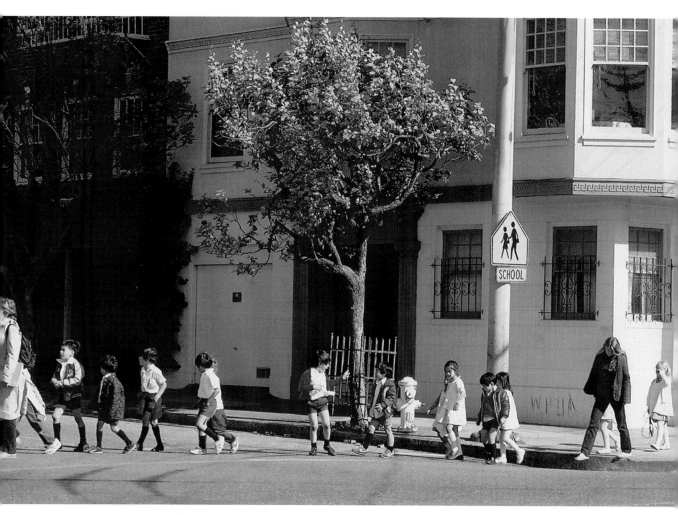

Always cross the street at the corner.

Watch Out for Cars and Bikes!

When you are walking, you are a **pedestrian**. Pedestrians need to look out for cars, trucks, and other moving **vehicles**.

If you need to cross the street, be sure to look both ways to see if a car is coming. You should do this even if you are crossing at a green light or a "Walk" sign. A car that is turning the corner might drive in front of you.

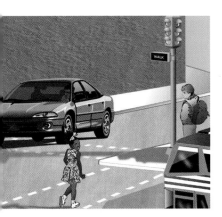

Watch traffic even when you're crossing with a green light.

When you are walking, you also need to watch for bikes. Because bicycles are quieter than cars, you might not hear them coming. If someone is riding their bike on the sidewalk or on a path in the park, stand still and let them pass.

Pedestrians need to watch out for cars.

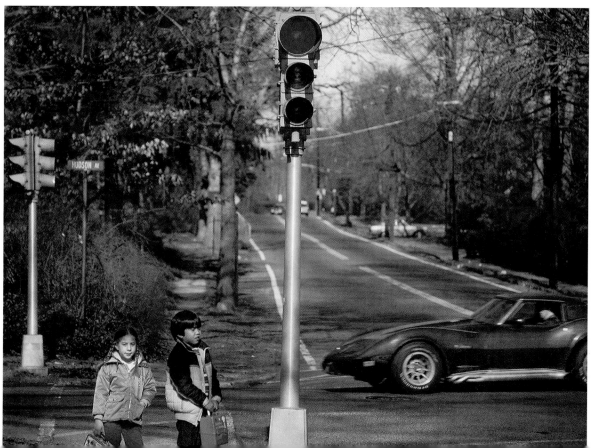

Railroad Tracks

Railroad tracks may look like fun places to play, but they are not! Many people have been hurt or killed walking or playing on railroad tracks.

A train cannot stop as fast as a car. That means that by the time the driver of the train sees you, it will be too late to stop the train. You might not be able to get off the tracks in time. You could also trip and fall on the tracks.

Stay back from the gate and tracks when the lights are flashing.

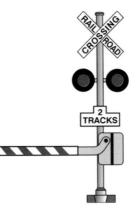

If you must cross railroad tracks, look both ways as you do when crossing the street. If the gates are down or the warning lights are flashing, stay back. Wait until the train passes. Never run in front of a train, even if it is stopped. You never know when the train might start moving again!

Never play on railroad tracks.

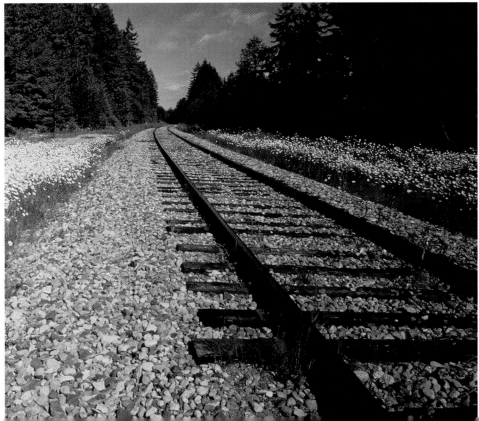

Staying Safe around Strangers

Cars, bikes, and trains aren't the only **dangerous** things in public places. Sometimes people can be dangerous, too.

The best way to protect yourself from a bully or a robber is to look **confident**. Walk quickly and steadily. Act like you know where you are going. Doing these things will make you seem strong. Bad people usually won't bother someone who appears strong and confident.

Another way to stay safe is to be aware of your surroundings. Try to avoid dangerous areas and empty buildings. Stay in busy places where there are lots of people. It's safe to walk with a friend— and it's fun, too!

Be alert when walking in a public place.

Don't Talk to Strangers

"Don't talk to strangers" is one of the most important safety rules. A **stranger** is anyone you don't know. A person could be a stranger even if he talks to you or acts friendly. A person could be a stranger even if she says she knows your parents or your friends.

Sometimes strangers will ask you for directions. If this happens to you, just say "I don't know" and walk away.

You should also walk away if a stranger offers you a ride home, asks if you want to see a new puppy or play a video game, or offers you candy or toys. Tell your parents what happened. If a stranger is hanging around your school or playground, tell a teacher.

Some neighborhoods have "safe houses." The people who live there will help children in trouble. A safe house has a sign in the window so you can identify it. You can always go to one of these houses for help.

There may be a safe house in your neighborhood.

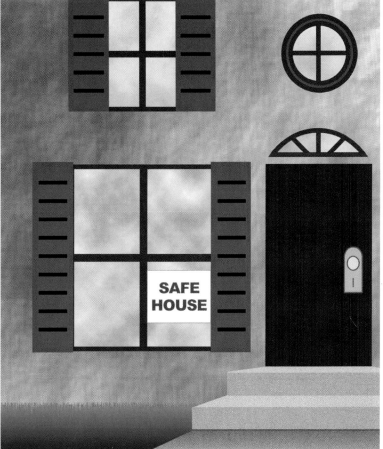

Keeping Your Things Safe

You should not only keep yourself safe, you should keep your things safe, too! The best way to keep other people from taking your things is to not show off. If you are wearing a nice necklace or watch, don't flash it around. If you are carrying money, don't tell anyone. Keep it in your pocket or backpack.

Bicycles can be stolen. You can keep your bike safe by locking it up. If you can't lock it, stay where you can see it. Don't drop your bike on the ground and run off to play. It might not be there when you get back!

Opposite page:
Always lock your bike when
you leave it unattended.

If anyone does try to take your money or your things, let the person have them. Nothing you own is worth getting hurt for. Sometimes giving in is the best way to stay safe.

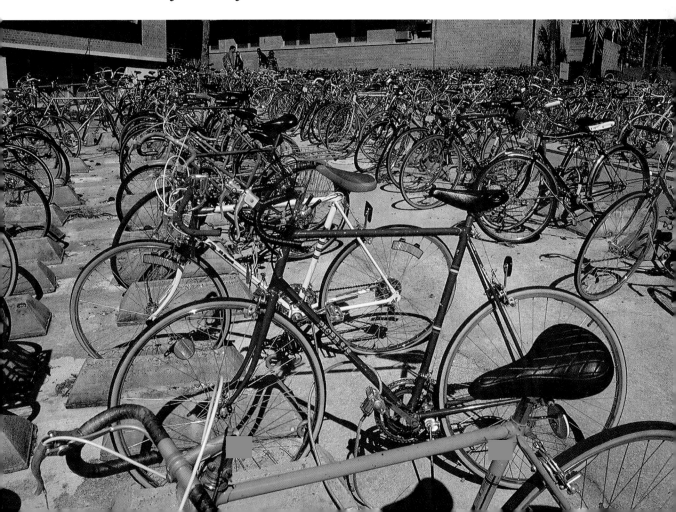

Elevators and Escalators

Before you step in, look at the people in the elevator. If you get a bad feeling about them, don't get on. You might look silly, but you will be safe!

If an elevator gets stuck, don't be scared. Push the "Alarm" button. The building **superintendent** or a police officer will come and help you. Many elevators have telephones to call 9-1-1.

Never climb out of an elevator or ride on the top of the car. Elevators are not safe places to play!

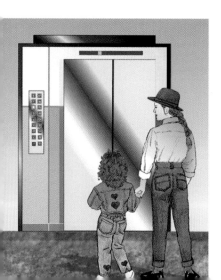

Never get in an elevator if you don't feel safe.

Escalators can also be **dangerous**. Never hang over the edge while you ride on one. Be careful not to let your coat or your sleeve get caught in the handrail. And don't run, or you might fall. That could hurt you—and other people, too!

Hold on to the handrail while riding an escalator.

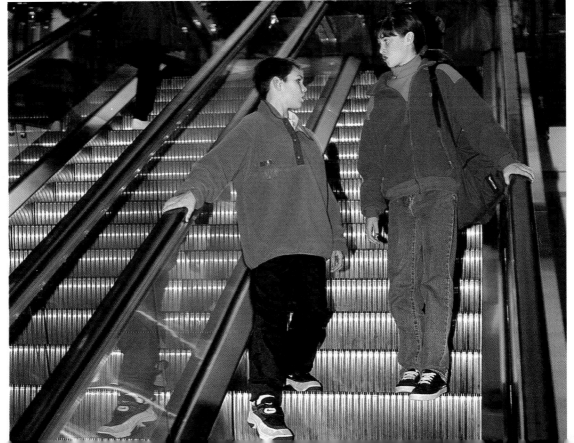

Asking for Help

There are many people in public places who can help if you get in trouble. The best person to ask is a police officer. A **crossing guard** or a mail carrier can also help you.

If you have problems in a store, look for a **security guard**. These people are easy to spot because they wear **uniforms**. Their job is to help people stay safe. If you can't find a security guard, ask a store clerk or cashier to help you. They will know what to do to help you put safety first!

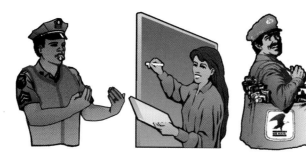

This page and opposite page: If you need help, look for helpers like these.

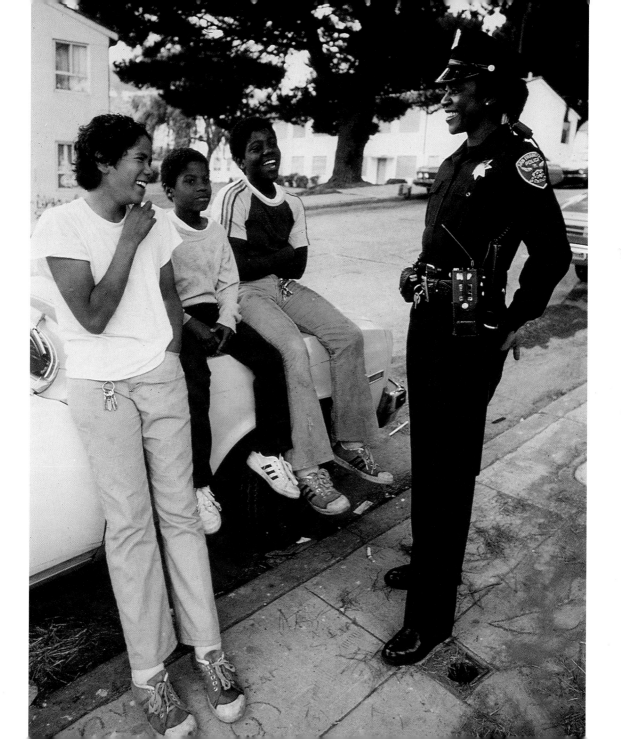

Glossary

Confident (KON-fuh-duhnt) - believing in your own abilities.

Crossing guard (KRAWSS-ing gard) - a person who stops traffic so people can cross the street.

Crosswalk (KRAWSS-wawk) - a place where it is safe to cross the street. A crosswalk is often marked with painted lines.

Dangerous (DAYN-jur-uhss) - likely to cause harm; not safe.

Intersection (IN-tur-sek-shuhn) - a place where two streets meet and cross each other.

Pedestrian (puh-DESS-tree-uhn) - someone who travels on foot.

Security guard (se-KURE-uh-tee gard) - a person who keeps people and objects safe.

Stranger (STRAYN-jur) - someone you do not know.

Superintendent (soo-pur-in-TEN-duhnt) - a person in charge of a building.

Uniform (YOO-nuh-form) - a special set of clothes worn by the members of a group or organization.

Vehicle (VEE-uh-kuhl) - something in which people or goods are carried from one place to another.

Internet Sites

Bicycling Safety
http://www.cam.org/~skippy/sites/cycling/SafetyLinks.html
Stories, studies, statistics, and tips on everything from safe cycling practices to maintenance. Special interest sections for kids and parents, and links to many interesting sites!

Safety Tips for Kids on the Internet
http://www.fbi.gov/kids/internet/internet.htm
The FBI has set up a "safety tips for the internet" website. It has very good information about how to protect yourself online.

National School Safety Center
http://www.nssc1.org/
This site provides training and resources for preventing school crime and violence.

Home Safety
http://www.safewithin.com/homesafe/
This site helps to make the home more secure, info on the health of the home environment and other safety resources.

These sites are subject to change.

Pass It On

Educate readers around the country by passing on information you've learned about staying safe. Share your little-known facts and interesting stories. Tell others about bike riding, school experiences, and any other stuff you'd like to discuss. We want to hear from you!

To get posted on the ABDO Publishing Company website E-mail us at **"adventure@abdopub.com"**

Download a free screen saver at www.abdopub.com

Index